£ι 99

12 LE.

FOR NL

SIMPLE STEPS TO INTE ___ι RHYTHMS,
ARRHYTHMIAS, BLOCKS, HYPERTROPHY, INFARCTS,
& CARDIAC DRUGS

By

AARON REED, MSN, CRNA

www.NurseMastery.com

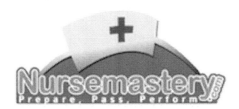

Copyright © 2015

1

INTRODUCTION

The 12 Lead EKG is frequently ordered as part of the cardiovascular assessment of patients in the hospital setting. The purpose of this book is to help nurses begin to understand and interpret EKG's, as well as the dynamic changes accompanying different pathological processes.

This book will help nursing students navigate course material and approach the NCLEX with a better understanding of electrophysiological principles. New graduate nurses can use this resource to grasp concepts that were skimmed over in nursing school and to help supplement cardiovascular assessments in the clinical setting.

Electrophysiology includes complex language that can be confusing and overwhelming. Some nursing students and new graduate nurses may purchase an advanced textbook, skim a few pages and never revisit the book again. Our hope in writing this book is to provide an understandable, yet comprehensive, approach to interpreting EKG's for the purpose of advancing through nursing school, passing the boards, and entering practice with a basic understanding of electrophysiology. We have tried to make this book as accessible and concise as possible. Repetition is necessary to build on what the nurse learns in this book. Progress toward mastery of this subject takes continual practice and repeated exposure to EKG's. This book will help the novice nurse grasp the rudimentary concepts and equip them to move forward in their practice.

This book will help the nurse break down the various sections of the EKG and its complexes. We will review what each part of the EKG represents and the abnormalities commonly associated with any deviations. *We will review changes resulting from arrhythmias, ischemia, injury, infarction, chamber enlargements, conduction blocks, and different drug and electrolyte disturbances*. Each type of arrhythmia will be explained followed by examples. Finally, we will share a comprehensive approach that combines all the important points of the previous chapters into a systematic approach to interpreting EKG's.

TABLE OF CONTENTS

THANK YOU FOR STUDYING WITH US!

<u>NURSEMASTERY.COM</u>

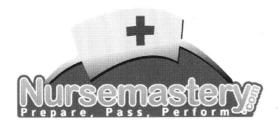

CHE
CKOUT:

"<u>NURSE NOTES</u>" APP: PATIENT TASK ALERTS

"<u>NCLEX REVIEW</u>" APP

<u>1000 NCLEX QUESTIONS eBOOK</u>

<u>75 NURSE CHEAT SHEETS eBOOK</u>

<u>SIGN UP FOR QUESTION OF THE DAY</u>

<u>Twitter</u>

<u>Youtube</u>

Facebook

FREE GIFT!

At NurseMastery.com/downloads

or

<u>Click link for 75 free NCLEX Questions & Cheat Sheets PDF</u>

CHAPTER 1. THE BASICS

The EKG is part of the cardiovascular examination. In isolation, the EKG can only provide discrete information. In order to make a complete diagnosis, the nurse must gather and evaluate several data sets, including:

- **Laboratory Data**

- **Physical Exam**

- **Health History**

- **X-ray**

- **EKG**

Incorporating knowledge of the physical status of the patient is essential. In the clinical setting, the nurse must be able to correlate EKG findings with the patient's appearance and complaints. For example, a patient may exhibit dominant S-waves in leads V5 or V6 with a dominant R-wave in V1. The nurse may suspect right ventricular hypertrophy but the diagnosis is made all the more easy if the patient presents with a complaint of shortness of breath as opposed to an ankle sprain.

The components of the cardiovascular examination and their interplay are important in interpreting the clinical presentation of the patient. Dysrhythmias, or arrhythmias, are disorders of the formation or conduction of the electrical impulses within the heart. Changes in the conduction of the heart may be evidenced by decreased pumping action of the heart, failure to deliver oxygenated blood, or decreased blood pressure, to name a few. Dysrhythmias are diagnosed by analyzing the EKG and named according to the site of origin of the impulse and the mechanism of formation or conduction involved.

The EKG is the recording of the heart's electrical activity, which is easily attainable and non-invasive. Like other muscles, the heart contracts in response to electrical depolarization of the muscle cells. The EKG reveals:

- **Rate**

- **Rhythm**

- **Chamber Enlargement**

- **Conduction Defects**

- **Ischemia**

- **Injury**

- **Infarct**

- **Signs of Drug & Electrolyte Disorders**

- Electrical Activity Related to Disease States

The EKG does NOT provide information about the mechanical activity of the heart. It can appear normal despite the presence of a pathological cardiac condition. EKG's must be correlated with the clinical situation and serial EKG's can be very useful.

ELECTROPHYSIOLOGY

All cardiac cells have the quality of *automaticity*, which is the ability to generate their own action potentials. The ability to spontaneously generate muscle contractions is a unique quality that allows the cardiac muscle to beat continuously without activation from nerves fibers. *Rhythmicity* is the ability to generate these potentials in a regular, repetitive manner. *Gap junctions* between cells allow the action potential from one cell to spread rapidly to all cells in the heart. This results in the heart acting as one large cell, in a sense. This coordination is necessary to mechanically pump blood in the proper sequence. Unfortunately, the electrical connectivity means that activation of any cell can inadvertently activate the heart as whole, which will be discussed later.

TERMS

Depolarization – Cells are electrically stimulated followed by mechanical contraction of myocardium.

Repolarization – Return of the cell's membrane potential to a resting state following depolarization.

The chambers are relaxed and re-filling in preparation to eject blood during the next contraction.

Leads – Looks at the electrical activity of the heart. Only 10 electrodes are used but at each level, voltage differences between two electrode points is measured and the combination of the two points is termed a "lead". This causes confusion because of the name "12-lead". For example, "lead I" is the voltage between the right arm electrode and the left arm electrode, whereas "lead II" is the voltage between the right arm and the left leg. In all combinations, the right leg electrode does not come into play because it provides a reference potential, or ground (neutral).

PRECORDIAL LEADS

The precordial (chest) leads each consist of a positive electrode placed on the chest of the patient. The precise position of each of the 6 precordial leads is important to provide an accurate EKG tracing.

V1 – 4th intercostal space, right sternal border.

V2 – 4th intercostal space, left sternal border.

V3 – Between leads V2 & V4.

V4 – 5th intercostal space, mid-clavicular line.

V5 – 5th intercostal space, anterior axillary line.

V6 – 5th intercostal space, mid-axillary line.

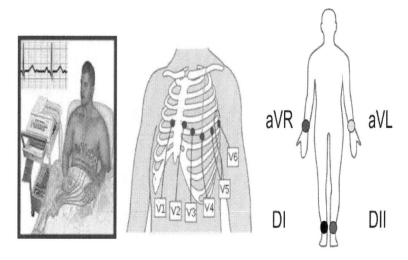

Credit: Jmarchn

PERFORMING 12-LEAD EKG

Position the patient supine, expose chest, and prepare skin. Place limb electrodes on large muscle groups with the RA (right arm) and LA (left arm) on the upper aspect of each arm. Place LL (left leg) and RL (right leg) on the medial aspect of each lower leg. Use the angle of Louis (notch in center of sternum) to begin counting the intercostal spaces as this angle is parallel with the 2nd rib. Each intercostal space is numbered for the rib above it. Respiratory variation and patient movement may create interference and compromise the clarity of the signal and accuracy of the information. Encourage the patient to be as still as possible.

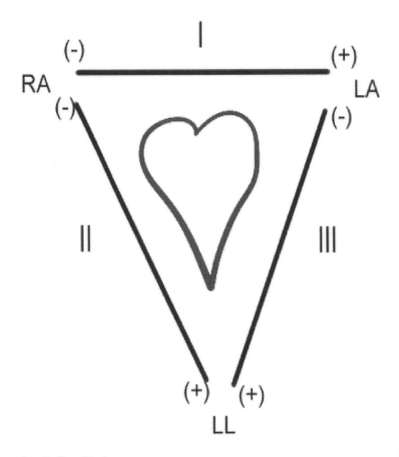

EKG leads are arranged into 2 planes. The frontal leads (lead I-III & aVR/aVF) view the heart from a vertical plane. The transverse leads (V1-V6) view the heart from a horizontal plane.

BIPOLAR LEADS

Bipolar refers to the use of two leads to develop a view of the heart. **Lead I** is arranged as a negative electrode placed on the right arm extending to the positive electrode on the left arm, creating a high lateral or superior view of the heart. **Lead II** is arranged as a negative electrode placed on the right arm extending to the positive electrode on the left leg, creating an inferior view of the heart. **Lead III** is arranged as a negative electrode placed on the left arm extending to the positive electrode placed on the left leg, creating an inferior view of the heart.

UNIPOLAR LEADS

These three leads view the heart from a positive electrode with the neutral point of reference in the center of the heart. A = augmented, V = voltage, followed by R, L, or F based on the placement. **aVR** is a positive electrode on the right arm known as the orphan lead because it is rarely used but can show left main coronary artery obstruction. **aVL** is a positive electrode on the left arm creating a high lateral or superior view of the wall of the heart. **aVF** is a positive electrode on the left foot creating an inferior view of the wall of the heart.

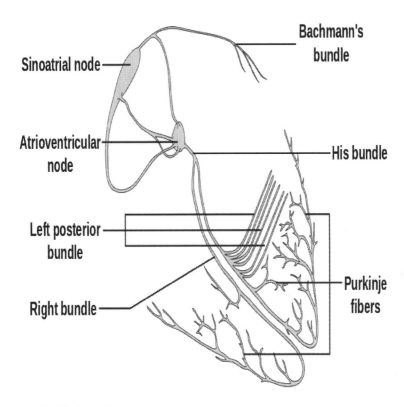

Sinoatrial node

Bachmann's bundle

Atrioventricular node

His bundle

Left posterior bundle

Right bundle

Purkinje fibers

Credit: Madhero88

CONDUCTION OF THE HEART

Electrical impulses originate in the sinoatrial node (**SA**), also known as the pacemaker, at a rate of 60-100 bpm.   The SA node is situated in the high right atrium (RA). The impulse is carried through the intra-atrial pathways and **Bachman's bundle** to the left atrium (LA) and right atrium (RA). The atria are separated from the ventricles by an electrically inert fibrous ring, which means that the only route of transmission of electrical depolarization from atria to ventricles is through the AV node. The impulse spreads through the atrioventricular node (**AV**) where it is slowed to ensure that the blood ejected from the atriums has filled the ventricles before contraction takes place. The AV node is also known as the back-up pacemaker because it fires at a rate of 40-60 bpm in situations when no impulse is initiated at the SA node. The impulse spreads down the **Bundle of HIS** to the left and right bundle systems and on to the **Purkinje fibers**. Overall, the septum is depolarized from left to right and depolarization occurs from the apex to the base of the heart. Repolarization occurs in the opposite direction.

It is critical to understand the heart's electrical conduction system. Pathology presented later in this book is dependent on an understanding of this circuitry. Bundle blocks, AV blocks, ectopic beats, and rhythm disturbances are directly related to aberrancy in normal conduction.

SUMMARY OF VIEWS OF THE HEART

Lead I = Left view

Lead II = Inferior view

Lead III = Inferior view

aVR = Right view

aVL = Left view

aVF = Inferior view

V1 & V2 = Right Ventricle

V3 & V4 = Septum

V5 & V6 = Left view

DETERMINING HR & MEASURING BOXES

Most monitors can print a calculated value or have a digital visual display. However, older methods help to convey and strengthen the concept. To calculate the heart rate, determine the time between two QRS complexes. The EKG has a grid with thick lines 5 mm apart (=0.2 seconds) and thin lines 1 mm apart (0.04 seconds). Therefore, 5 big boxes between each QRS complex is 60 beats per minute, 3 is 100 bpm, and 2 is 150 bpm.

The **square counting method** is ideal for regular heart rates. Use the sequence 300-150-100-75-60-50. Count from the first QRS complex that is intersected by a thick line as 300, the next thick line as 150, and so on. Counting down sequentially stops at the next QRS complex. When the second QRS complex is between two lines, take the average of the two numbers from the sequence. For example, if the next QRS complex lands between the 5th and 6th big boxes, the average would be 55 bpm.

The **calculator method** involves counting the small (1 mm) squares between two QRS complexes. The

EKG paper runs at a rate of 25 mm/sec. As such: HR = ((25 mm/sec x 60 sec/min) / number of squares) OR **(1500 / number of squares).** This method is ideal for tachycardia.

The **3-second marker method** is used with non-regular rhythms. Count the number of QRS complexes that fit into 3 seconds and multiply this number by 20 to find the number of beats per minute.

Sinus Bradycardia is a heart rate below 60 bpm. Bradycardia can be caused by:

- Hypothermia

- Vagal stimulation (cough, bearing down)

- Hypothyroidism

- Beta-blockers (metoprolol, etc.)

- Increased intracranial pressure

- Ischemia

Sinus Tachycardia is a heart rate above 100 bpm. Tachycardia can be caused by:

- Pain

- Fever

- Thyrotoxicosis → excess of thyroid hormone

- Hypovolemia

- Vagolytic drugs (atropine)

- Anemia

- Emotional excitability

P-WAVE

Represents atrial depolarization and is the first positive deflection on the EKG. The wave should be rounded and not notched. Height < 2.5 – 3 mm with a width < 0.11 seconds. The P-wave is upright in leads I, II, aVF, & V4 – 6, inverted in aVR, and variable in III, V1 – 3.

PR-INTERVAL/SEGMENT

Represents a short, physiological delay as the atrioventricular (AV) node slows the electrical depolarization before it proceeds to the ventricles. The delay is responsible for the PR-interval, a short period when no electrical activity is seen on EKG. Normal length is 0.12 - .20 seconds or 120 – 200 ms (milliseconds), which is represented by 3 -5 small boxes on EKG paper. It is measured from the beginning of the P-wave to the first deflection of the QRS complex. PR-segment is isoelectric and is measured from the end of the P-wave to the first deflection of the QRS complex.

QRS-Complex

Represents ventricular depolarization, which is usually the largest part of the EKG signal due to the large muscle mass of the ventricles. The complex takes on different shapes depending on the lead and axis. Length is 0.06 - 0.12 or 60 – 120 ms, which is represented by 3 small boxes on EKG paper. It is measured from the first deflection of the QRS complex to the end of the QRS complex at the isoelectric line. Several sequences and combinations of waves of the QRS can be seen but typically, the Q-wave is the first initial downward, or negative, deflection. The R-wave is the next upward deflection. The S-wave is the final deflection downwards. The QRS is positive in leads that look at the left side of the heart, negative in leads that look at the right side of the heart, biphasic in leads V3 – 4, and negative in aVR.

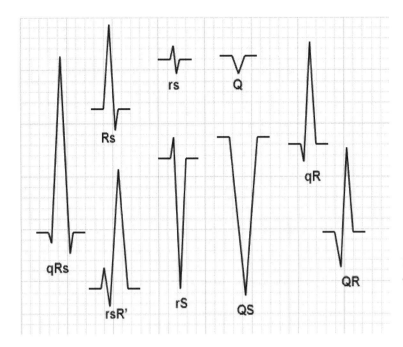

ST-SEGMENT

Represents the interval between ventricular depolarization and repolarization. It should be isoelectric (even with baseline) and then curve into the T-wave.

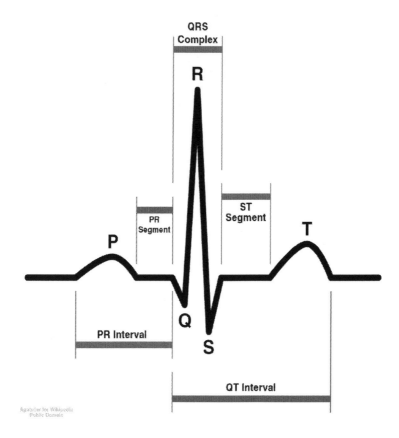

Credit: Hank Van Helvete

T-WAVE

Represents ventricular repolarization. It should project in the same direction as the QRS in leads I, II, III, aVF, & V3 – 4. It is negative in aVR and variable in V1 – V2.

QT-INTERVAL

It spans from the beginning of the QRS to the end of the T-wave and should be 0.35 – 0.45 seconds. The QT becomes shorter as the heart rate increases. Commonly, the QT should be < ½ the R – R interval. Prolonged QT-intervals can result from congenital abnormalities, antidysrhythmics, tricyclic antidepressants, MI/ischemia, Sub-arachnoid hemorrhage, electrolyte disturbances, anti-emetics (Zofran), and Amiodarone/Haldol/Procainamide.

Q-WAVE

A Q-wave is any negative deflection that precedes an R-wave. *Small* Q-waves are normal in most leads. If they are > 1 mm wide, > 2 mm deep, > 25% of the QRS complex, or seen in leads V1 – 3, they are considered pathologic. They usually indicate current or prior myocardial infarction.

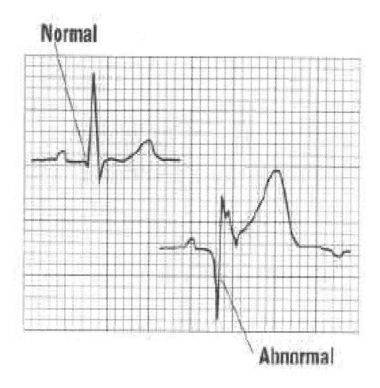

Normal

Abnormal

RHYTHMS

Sinus Rhythm

- Rhythm: Regular (same distance between R-waves)

- Rate: 60 – 99 bpm

- QRS duration: Normal

- P-wave: Seen before each QRS-complex

- PR-interval: Normal (< 5 small boxes)

Supraventricular   Tachycardia (SVT)

24

- Rhythm: Regular

- Rate: 140 – 220 bpm

- QRS duration: Typically normal

- P-wave: Hidden by T-wave

- PR-interval: Varies d/t site of SVT pacemaker

- Note: Abnormal narrow complex tachycardia with impulse that originates in the aria but is not properly controlled by the SA node.

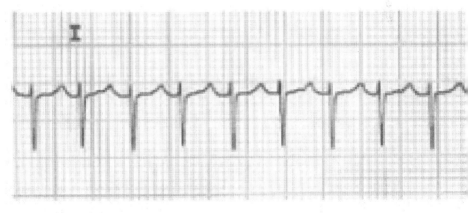

Atrial Fibrillation

- Rhythm: Irregularly irregular

- Rate: 100 – 170 bpm

- QRS duration: Typically normal

- P-wave: Random firing makes indistinguishable

- PR-interval: Not   measurable

25

- Note: Impulses generated from multiple sites creating irregular impulses to the ventricles that stimulate irregular heartbeats. Associated with palpitations, fainting, or chest pain. Presents risk of poor propulsion of blood from atria leading to emboli formation that could enter pulmonary circulation.

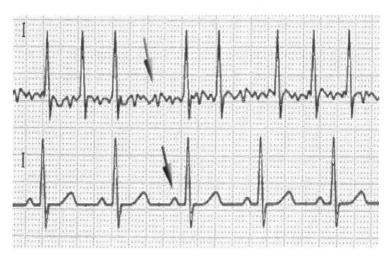

Atrial Flutter

- Rhythm: Regular

- Rate: Approx. 100-120 bpm

- QRS duration: Typically normal

- P-wave: Saw-tooth flutter waves at 2:1 or 3:1 ratio

- P-wave rate: 300 bpm

- PR-interval: Not measured

- Note: Atrial impulses are generating a rapid heart rate without involvement of the AV node.

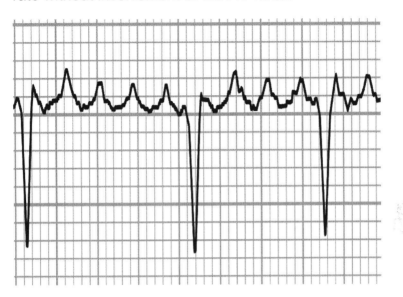

Premature Atrial Complex (PAC)

- Rhythm: Regular

- Rate: Normal

- QRS: Normal, absent, wide, or RBBB in appearance

- P-wave: Inverted, hidden in preceding T-wave

- PR-interval: May be prolonged

- Note: Premature impulses arising from atria that are captured by the ventricles, producing a beat. Several features may be present including: abnormal P-wave followed by normal QRS, P-wave hidden in preceding T-wave (produces peaked T-wave), shorter or longer

27

PR-intervals, RBBB appearance (right bundle branch block appearance producing widened QRS or double-notched R-wave), or P-wave not followed by QRS. Pictured below is a normal beat in each lead followed by an example of a PAC.

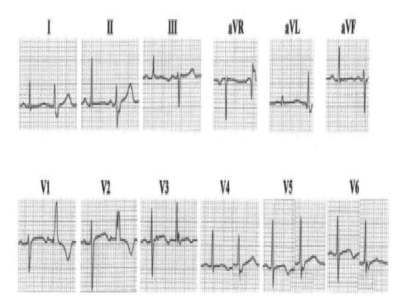

Premature Ventricular Complexes (PVC)

- Rhythm: Regular

- Rate: Normal

- QRS duration: Normal, sometimes wide

- P-wave ratio: 1:1

- P-wave rate: Normal according to QRS rate

- PR-interval: Normal

- Note: A portion of the heart depolarizes sooner than it should from a signal within the ventricles creating wide QRS-like waveforms. When multiple PVC's appear similar it is termed **Unifocal** (originating from same location). When they appear different, they are termed **Multifocal** (originating from different locations). When PVC's occur every other beat it is termed **Bigeminy**. Every 3rd beat is termed **Trigeminy**.

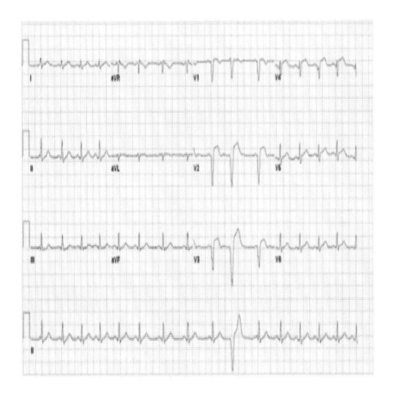

Junctional Rhythm

- Rhythm: Regular

- Rate: 40 – 60 bpm

- QRS duration: Normal

- P-wave ratio: 1:1, sometime *not visible* or inverted

- P-wave rate: Same as QRS

- PR-interval: Variable

- Note: Sinoatrial node no longer controls rhythm as the AV node takes over, resulting in a slower rate.

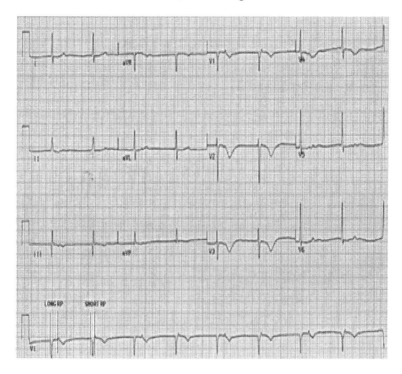

Atrial & Ventricular Pacing

- Rhythm: Regular or   Irregular

- Rate: 60 – 99 bpm

- QRS: Prolonged with Ventricular pacing

- P-wave: Prolonged with Atrial pacing

- Note: Pacemakers are devices used when electrical impulses are not conducting properly within the heart. Pacemakers produce visually apparent *spikes* on the EKG preceding either the P-wave or QRS complex as the device produces electrical impulses to stimulate a mechanical response from the heart. The external or internal device may pace periodically or continuously in the atria, ventricles, or both. They are typically used for bradyarrhythmias. Pictured below is ventricular pacing. The device fails to pace the atria toward the end of the strip as evidenced by a pacer spike without a subsequent P-wave.

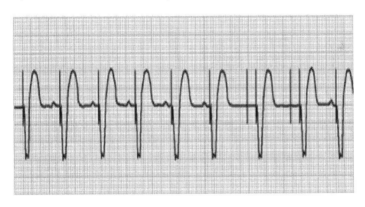

Ventricular Tachycardia (VT)

- Rhythm: Regular

- Rate: 170 – 190 bpm

31

- QRS duration: Prolonged

- P-wave: Not visible

- Note: Ventricles generate irregular, rapid rhythm. This is a life-threatening rhythm that leads to cardiac arrest. It requires defibrillation to quickly re-set and reorganize the electrical activity of the heart.

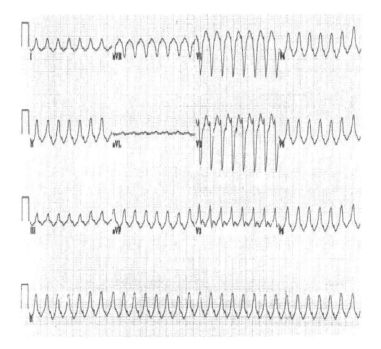

Ventricular Fibrillation (VF)

- Rhythm: Irregular

- Rate: > 300 bpm

- QRS duration: Undetectable

32

- P-wave: Undetectable

- Note: Defibrillation is required immediately as cardiac output is essentially non-existent due to the heart essentially quivering with sporadic electrical activity that is completely disorganized.

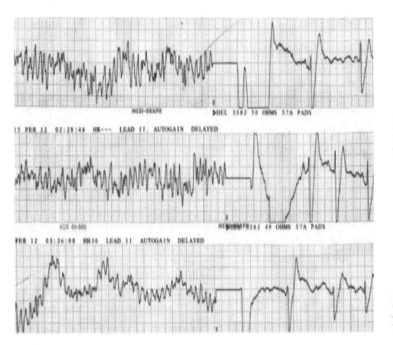

Asystole

- Rhythm: None

- Rate: 0 bpm

- QRS duration: None

- P-wave: None

- Note: Non-shockable, begin CPR.

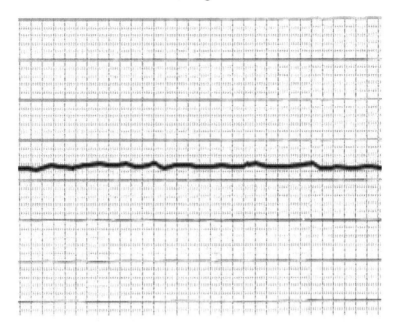

CHAPTER 2. ISCHEMIA, INJURY, INFARCT

Decreased blood supply through the coronary arteries to the myocardium leads to a lack of oxygen, also known as ischemia. With **ischemia**, ST-segment depression or T-wave inversion is seen on EKG. **Injury** results from prolonged ischemia and is evidenced by ST-segment elevation. Death of tissue, or **infarction**, may or may not produce a pathologically deep Q-wave. EKG changes are seen in leads over the affected area.

Acute coronary syndrome refers to a group of conditions resulting from lack of blood flow in the coronary arteries. The most common cause is ruptured plaque and the most common symptom is chest pain. This condition exists on a continuum, meaning that secondary chest pain can range from stable to unstable. **Unstable angina** occurs at rest, usually lasts 3 – 5 minutes, is severe and of new onset, and worsens over time. The reduction of coronary blood due to transient platelet aggregation results in unstable plaque, which can break off or totally occlude certain branches. **Stable angina** has a more solid fibrous cap and only develops with activity or stress.

CORONARY VASCULATURE

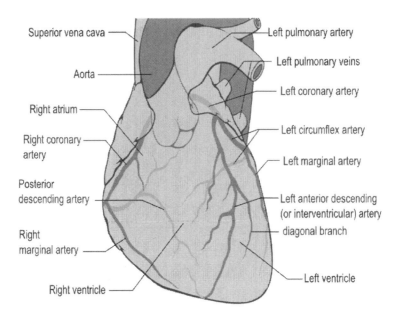

Superior vena cava

Aorta

Right atrium

Right coronary artery

Posterior descending artery

Right marginal artery

Right ventricle

Left pulmonary artery

Left pulmonary veins

Left coronary artery

Left circumflex artery

Left marginal artery

Left anterior descending (or interventricular) artery

diagonal branch

Left ventricle

Left main artery: Provides blood supply to the left side of the heart. Also known as the "widow-maker" because of the large amount of myocardial tissue supplied by this artery.

Left anterior descending: Provides blood supply to the left ventricle and anterior 2/3 of the *septum* (wall dividing left from right side of heart). Also supplies the right bundle branch and both the anterior and posterior fascicles of the left bundle branch.

Circumflex: Provides blood supply to the lateral wall of the left ventricle, left atrium, 40-50% of the SA node, 10% of the AV node, and posterior fascicle.

Right coronary artery: Provides blood supply to the right atrium and ventricle, posterior fascicle, 50-60%

of the SA node, 90% of the AV node, and posterior 1/3 of the septum.

ISCHEMIA

Refers to a decrease in blood flow to the myocardium due to narrowed coronary arteries. Ischemia can also result from a mismatch between oxygen supply and demand during periods of stress when the heart is tachycardic or pumps against increased resistance (hypertension, systemic vascular resistance, aortic stenosis, increased peripheral vascular resistance, etc.). Ischemia leads to **abnormal repolarization** but can be reversible.

Early EKG changes secondary to ischemia include peaked T-waves followed by deep T-wave inversion as the situation worsens over time.

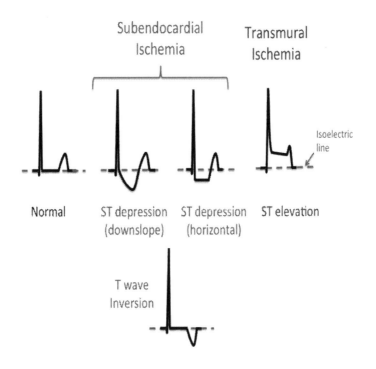

T-wave changes can also occur in **Bundle Branch Blocks** (cessation of conduction of electrical impulses beyond a portion of the Bundle of HIS), **pericarditis** (inflammation of the fibrous sac surrounding the heart), **hypertrophic cardiomyopathy** (reduced myocardial blood flow resulting from enlarged myocardium pressing outward and against the coronary arteries situated along the surface of the heart), **hyperkalemia** (increased potassium), or **subarachnoid hemorrhage** (area between arachnoid membrane and pia mater surrounding brain).

ST-segment depression is another electrical signal of the heart suffering from ischemia. ST-segment depression is below the isoelectric line and 0.04 seconds after the **J-point** (point where the QRS complex meets the ST-segment). ST-segment depression can be down-sloping or horizontal.

INJURY

Myocardial injury results from prolonged ischemia. This represents a serious threat because abnormal depolarization occurs, affecting the hearts ability to pump blood. EKG changes include elevated ST-segment > 0.04 sec after the J-point, which is cove-shaped in nature.

Injuries can result from a variety of causes. **Prinzmetal angina** is characterized by ST-segment elevation with chest pain due to temporary coronary artery vasospasms. **Ventricular aneurysms** are confirmed by echocardiogram (non-invasive ultrasound test to visualize heart structures) and physical exam when persistent ST-segment elevation occurs after infarct (tissue death, which creates an outward bulging at site of injury). **Left main disease/three vessel disease** presents as ST-segment depression with ST-elevation in aVR and V1.

INFARCT

Infarct results in necrosis of tissue due to death of muscle cells. Previous, or old, infarcts present with pathological **Q-waves** > 0.04 seconds and 25% of the height of the R-wave. Q-waves are the result of the absence of electrical activity from scar tissue. They usually take several hours to days to develop. They usually persist indefinitely. Lead III often shows Q-waves, which are not pathologic unless Q-waves are also seen in lead II and aVF.

EVOLUTION OF ACUTE MI

The earliest sign of a myocardial infarction is a hyperacute T-wave followed by ST-segment elevation, T-wave inversion, and Q-wave formation.

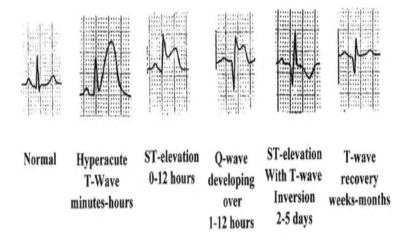

Normal	Hyperacute T-Wave minutes-hours	ST-elevation 0-12 hours	Q-wave developing over 1-12 hours	ST-elevation With T-wave Inversion 2-5 days	T-wave recovery weeks-months

The ST-segment returns to baseline. T-wave inversion persists and may deepen while Q-waves remain. The T-wave becomes upright eventually. This is also known as **STEMI** (ST-elevation MI)

NSTEMI (non-ST-elevation MI) presents as ST-depression and T-wave inversion. No progression to

Q-wave exists so this can also be called a **non-Q-wave** myocardial infarction. Diagnosis is made based on history and clinical markers. This situation may pose a risk of re-infarction.

Anterior MI's refer to the sight of injury. Looking at specific leads can narrow the location further. Anterior MI's are identified in leads V2- V4. Anterior septal MI's are seen in leads V1 – V2 as a result of septal branch occlusions. When the **LAD** (left anterior descending artery) or Diagonal is involved, changes will be seen in leads V3 – V4. The changes that are seen include ST-segment elevation, deep Q-waves, & loss of **R-wave progression** (V1 should show small R-waves which then become larger through precordial leads and largest in V4 before becoming small in V6 again). Anterior MI's can lead to heart failure, shock, atrial & ventricular dysrhythmias, **Mobitz II** (intermittent, non-conducted P-waves without progressive prolongation of PR-interval), complete heart block (CHB), BBB, ventricular septal defect (VSD), rupture, or aneurysm.

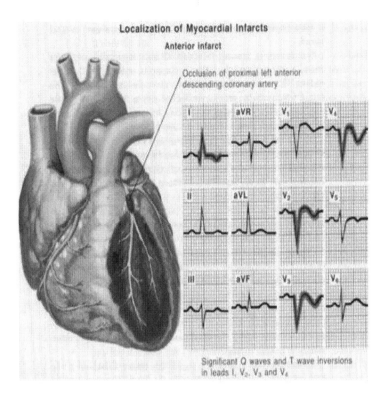

Localization of Myocardial Infarcts

Anterior infarct

Occlusion of proximal left anterior descending coronary artery

Significant Q waves and T wave inversions in leads I, V₂, V₃ and V₄

Inferior MI's are seen in leads II, III, and aVF with ST-segment elevation and Q-waves. Reciprocal changes include ST-segment depression in leads I and aVL. Inferior MI's involve occlusion of the **RCA** (right coronary artery) or **Circumflex** (LCx). This condition can result in bradyarrhythmias, **Mobitz I** (PR-interval lengthens progressively until the atrial impulse is blocked and doesn't produce a QRS), and AIVR (accelerated idioventricular rhythm, a regular rhythm when vagal tone exceeds sympathetic tone resulting in a ventricular pacemaker that overrides the sinus node with a HR of 50-100 bpm)

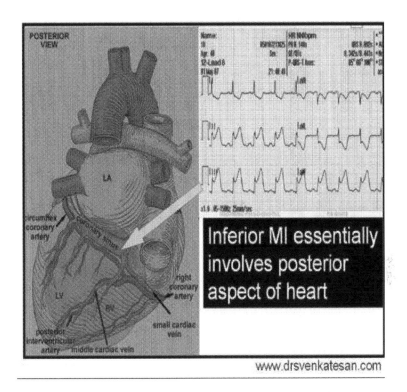

Inferior MI essentially involves posterior aspect of heart

www.drsvenkatesan.com

Right Ventricular Infarcts have characteristics similar to inferior MI's in that ST-elevation in II, III, and aVF are present. If ST-segment elevation in V1 and depression in V2 are present, suspect right ventricular infarction in the setting of an inferior MI. RV infarctions complicate up to 40% of inferior STEMI's. Patients with RV infarctions are very preload (blood returning to right side of heart) sensitive due to poor contractility and can develop severe hypotension in response to nitrates. Hypotension is usually treated with fluid loading. Symptoms include elevated **JVP** (jugular vein distension from build up of fluid on right side of heart) and weak pulse. Potential

43

complications are **AV block** (impairment of
conduction between atria and ventricles resulting in
1st degree, 2nd degree, 3rd degree block), hypotension,
and dependent filing pressures.

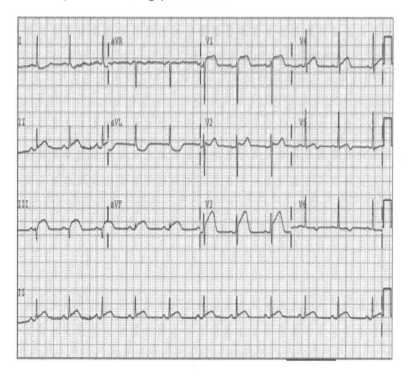

Lateral Wall MI's are shown as ST-elevation on
leads I, aVL, V5 – V6 with ST-segment depression in
IIII and aVF. It is usually part of a larger anterolateral
STEMI. The lateral wall of the LV is supplied by
branches of the LAD and LCx. Complications include
PVC's (premature ventricular complexes, which is an
early beat arising from the ventricles that looks wide
and interrupts the P-wave) and LV dysfunction.

Posterior Wall MI's are the mirror image of anterior MI's. This is because a standard EKG does not have a direct view of the back of the heart. Tall, broad R-waves are seen in V1– 3 along with horizontally depressed ST-segments and upright T-waves. Posterior wall infarctions involve the LCx and RCA. Complications include PVC's, AV block, and LV dysfunction. Posterior wall infarctions may be extensions of lateral and inferior MI's.

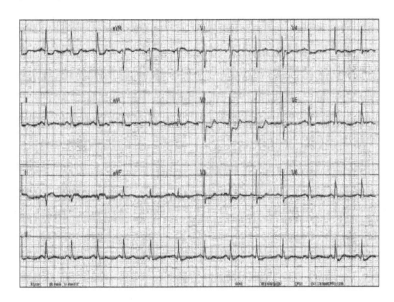

Pericarditis is an inflammation of the sac surrounding the heart. The patient may feel chest pain on inspiration. A friction rub can sometimes be auscultated. Pericarditis is characterized by diffuse ST-segment elevation and **PR-segment depression** in leads I, II, III, aVF, V2 – 6.

REVIEW

Ischemia = inverted T-waves, depressed ST-segment

Acute injury = ST-elevation

Infarct = Q-waves

Overview of Infarcts

Location of Infarct	Arterial Supply	Indicative Changes	Reciprocal Changes
Anterior	LAD	**V1-V4**	II, III, aVF
Inferior	RCA	**II, III, aVF**	I, aVL
Lateral	Circumflex	I, aVL, V5, V6	V1
Posterior	Posterior Descending (RCA)	None	V1, V2
Septal	Septal Perforating (LAD) Posterior Descending (RCA	Loss of R wave in V1, V2, or V3	None

CHAPTER 3. CARDIAC ENLARGEMENT

Chamber enlargement can occur in both the atria and ventricles. When one or more chambers in the heart increase in size it is usually due to an increase in pressure or volume. Echocardiogram and physical examination will confirm diagnosis. Enlargement can also be referred to as **hypertrophy**, which is when the heart muscle becomes thicker. Left ventricular hypertrophy is caused by an increase in left ventricular workload, e.g., aortic valve stenosis or hypertension. Right ventricular hypertrophy is caused by an increase in right ventricular workload e.g., pulmonary emboli or emphysema.

Left atrial enlargement can be identified in lead II as a broad notched upright "P". Since the P-wave originates in the atrium, this is where to look for the defect. In V1, the P-wave will dip below the isoelectric line. Left atrial hypertrophy can be caused by mitral stenosis, LVH, or left ventricular dysfunction.

Left Atrial Enlargement

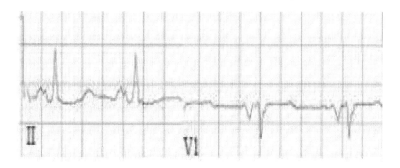

Right atrial enlargement is also seen in leads II and
V1. In lead II, there will be a tall, peaked P-wave.
Pulmonale coincidentally starts with a "P" as well,
making it easy to remember as a cause of this
condition. In V1, there will be a tall upstroke of the
initial P-wave or a slightly negative deflection below
baseline. Right atrial hypertrophy can be caused by
severe lung disease, pulmonary stenosis, RV failure,
and tricuspid stenosis.

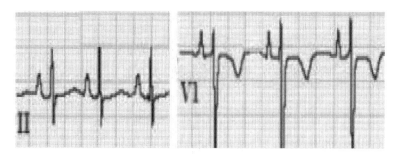

Left ventricular hypertrophy causes a widening of
the QRS to 0.12 seconds, especially evident in leads
V1 – V6. The S-wave in V1 or V2 is deepened and

the R-wave in V4-6 is taller. ST-depression can sometimes be seen in lead V5 – V6, also known as a strain pattern. LVH can be caused by hypertension, aortic stenosis, cardiomyopathy, aortic regurgitation, or mitral regurgitation.

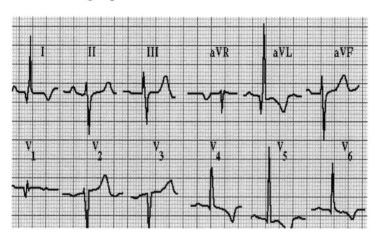

Right ventricular hypertrophy manifests as widening of the QRS, dominant R-wave in V1, and dominant S-wave in V5 or V6. Right ventricular strain pattern can be seen in V1 & 2 as ST-segment depression and T-wave inversion as well as ST-segment elevation and upright T-wave in V5 – 6. Right ventricular enlargement is caused by pulmonary hypertension, pulmonary stenosis, pulmonary embolism, or chronic lung disease.

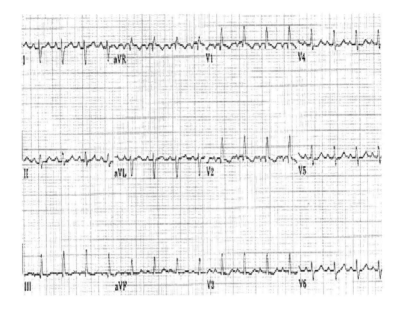

REVIEW

LAE = Notched P-wave lead II, deep P-wave in V1

RAE = Peaked P-wave lead II & V1

LVE = Widened QRS, deep S-wave in V1 or V2, peaked R-wave in V4 - 6, ST-depression.

RVE = Widened QRS, peaked R-wave V1, deep S-wave V5 – 6.

CHAPTER 4. CONDUCTION DEFECTS

Conduction defects can be identified on EKG as blocks or delays in the normal conduction pattern of the heart. In order to maximize the efficiency of cardiac contractions and cardiac output, the conduction system must create a delay between the contractions of the atria and ventricles, begin contractions at the apex of the heart to eject blood into the great arteries, and allow relaxation to give the heart an opportunity to fill up again.

AV BLOCKS

First-degree blocks create a conduction delay that *prolongs* the PR-interval > 200 ms (5 small boxes, normally 0.12-0.2 sec.). The most common causes of AV blocks are AV nodal disease, enhanced vagal tone (well trained athletes), myocarditis, acute MI, and electrolyte disturbances. Medications that contribute include CCB's, BB's, cardiac glycosides, and digitalis.

Second degree, Mobitz I (Wenckebach) is characterized by a *progressive prolongation* of the PR-interval until a QRS is dropped (not conducted/absent from strip). The P-to-P interval remains mostly *constant*. The ratio of P:QRS tends to repeat itself at approximately 3:2, 4:3, or 5:4. This is almost always a benign condition but when symptomatic, the patient may require atropine to improve conduction.

51

Second degree, Mobitz II presents as *intermittent* non-conducted QRS complexes *without* progressive prolongation of the PR-interval. The PR-interval remains constant. This rhythm may quickly progress to a complete heart block and significant bradycardia. It is most often caused by an anterior MI, idiopathic fibrosis, valve repair surgery, myocarditis, lupus, amyloidosis, hyperkalemia, BB's, CCB's, or digoxin. Treatment includes transcutaneous pacing and atropine based on severity of symptoms.

Third-degree (complete) ceases any AV node conduction between the atria and ventricles. Syncope and sudden cardiac death are serious threats. Since the electrical stimulation is originating from each area independently, the atrial rate is approx. 100 bpm and the ventricular rate is approx. 40 bpm. There is a complete dissociation between atrial P-waves and ventricular QRS complexes. Many antihypertensive, antianginal, antiarrhythmic, and heart failure medications can cause this condition and must be discontinued. In most cases, atropine will have no effect so temporary pacing (external, artificial electrical stimulation) as a bridge to permanent, internal pacemaker implantation is often necessary.

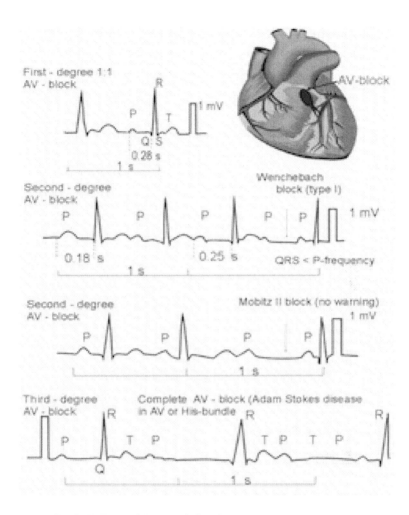

First - degree 1:1
AV - block

Second - degree
AV - block

Second - degree
AV - block

Third - degree
AV - block

AV-block

Wenchebach
block (type I)

QRS < P-frequency

Mobitz II block (no warning)

Complete AV - block (Adam Stokes disease
in AV or His-bundle

BUNDLE BRANCH BLOCKS

Bundle branch blocks (BBB) are characterized as
cessation of conduction through the left or right
bundle causing a delay in conduction of the ventricles.
Widening of the QRS > 0.12 seconds is seen, as well
as secondary ST and T-wave changes. Normal
conduction depolarizes the septum from left to right,

53

then inferior to superior. When a bundle branch or fascicle becomes injured (infarct, scarring) it can cease to conduct electrical impulses correctly. In the event that electrical impulses can no longer use the regular pathways, they may shift through muscle fibers, which slows movement and changes the direction of the impulse. Ventricular asynchrony and cardiac output may drop.

Left bundle branch block reverses the normal direction of septal depolarization so that it now becomes right to left. The impulse is forced to spread to the RV first, then the LV via the right bundle branch. Consequently, the QRS is elongated beyond 0.12 seconds and the Q-wave is missing. *Tall, double-notched R-waves* appear in leads I, aVL, and V5 – 6. Deep S-waves are seen in V1 – 3. The notch is the result of the ventricles not being activated simultaneously, but sequentially, resulting in 2 small peaks at the top of the R-wave instead of just 1. This condition can result from hypertension, aortic stenosis, anterior MI, dilated cardiomyopathy, ischemic heart disease, digoxin toxicity, or hyperkalemia. LBBB requires a cardiac evaluation so that those with syncope can be worked up for pacemakers. Biventricular pacemakers may help synchronize heart contractions better.

Left bundle branch block characteristics

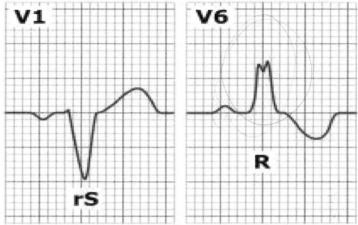

Right bundle branch block characteristics

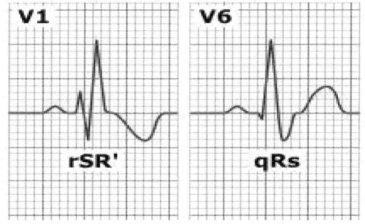

Right bundle branch blocks are characterized by a delay in activation of the right ventricle as depolarization spreads across the septum from the left ventricle. Since the left ventricle in activated in the usual fashion, the initial portion of the QRS looks the same but is widened. The delay of the right ventricle creates an *additional R-wave* seen in leads V1 – 3 and a *deep, wide S-waves* in leads I and V6. Secondary ST-segment & T-wave changes include depression and inversion. RBBB can be congenital or a consequence of heart disease. Patients may be entirely asymptomatic. However, if the block is diffuse or associated with further ventricular damage, a pacemaker may be needed.

WOLFF-PARKINSON-WHITE SYNDROME (WPW)

Wolff-Parkinson-White Syndrome patients are prone to re-entry tachycardia due to congenital accessory pathways. **Accessory pathways** are additional electrical conduction pathways between two parts of the heart that alter the conduction system. There is a small risk of sudden cardiac death associated with this condition. Pre-excitation occurs when the ventricles are activated too early as electrical impulses bypass the **AV node** through an accessory pathway. When the atria are experiencing fibrillation or flutter, a tachyarrhythmia may occur.

Orthodromic tachycardia refers to conduction that passes through the AV node (normal direction) and then back through the accessory pathway resulting in a shortened PR-interval and narrow QRS.

Antidromic tachycardia refers to conduction that passes through the accessory pathway first (opposite of normal) and then back through the AV node resulting in a **Delta Wave** (slurring, gradual upstroke of the QRS) and a wide QRS.

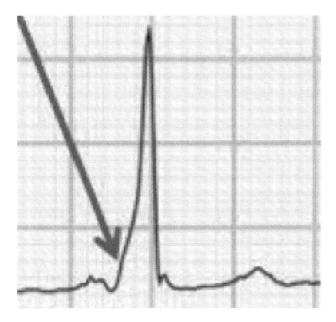

WPW Sinus rhythm will display EKG features similar to that of antidromic tachycardia but without the high heart rate. Note the delta waves.

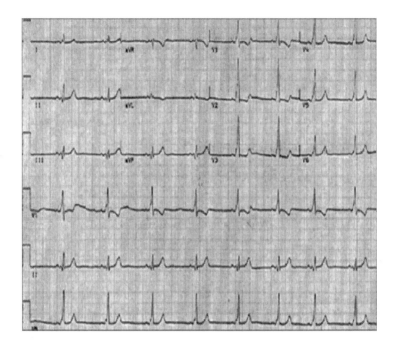

Chapter 5. Drug & Electrolyte

EKG changes are often times associated with imbalances in electrolytes and medications. Distinctive patterns can be seen, especially with patients experiencing potassium and calcium disturbances. Medications like Digoxin can also display distinct patterns that are recognizable to the trained nurse. Identifying and treating these pathological conditions is important to the patient's health. As always, these findings must be correlated with a thorough clinical examination, health history, and further diagnostic studies to confirm a diagnosis.

Potassium plays a major role in maintaining the integrity of the cardiac **myocyte** (heart muscle cell). Depolarization requires the exchange of both potassium and calcium ions across the cell membrane. Alterations in the concentration can affect the heart's electrical activity and EKG pattern. Potassium is the most plentiful intracellular **cation** (positively charged electrolyte). The intracellular fluid (**ICF**) concentration is 150 – 160 mEq/L, while the extracellular fluid (**ECF**) concentration is 3.5 – 4.5 mEq/L. Changes in the ratio between ICF and ECF concentrations can have evident effects on the heart.

HYPOKALEMIA

Potassium is excreted in the urine, feces, and through perspiration.

Hypokalemia is commonly seen with vomiting, diarrhea, prolonged diuretic use, and nasogastric suctioning. Hypokalemia results in exaggerated **U-waves** (additional hump that looks like extra T-wave), ST-segment depression, and flat T-waves. Smooth muscle atony and cardiac arrhythmias are common, including: bradycardia, AV block, and atrial tachycardia. The underlying cause/s of hypokalemia should be identified and corrected. Acid-base correction, oral or IV potassium replacement, and prevention of further loss are all important interventions.

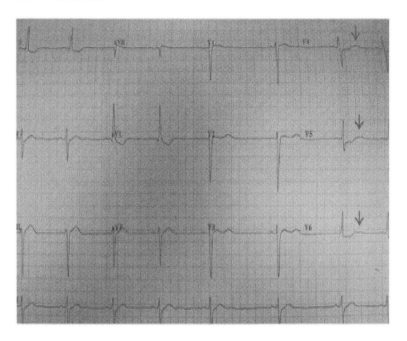

HYPERKALEMIA

Hyperkalemia can be caused by acute renal failure, potassium sparing diuretics (spironolactone, etc.), or acidosis. The most common EKG finding is tall, **peaked T-waves** with a flattened P-wave and a widened QRS. Hyperkalemia can cause a range of symptoms from neuromuscular irritability to loss of muscle tone. The underlying cause must be identified and corrected. Insulin administered with glucose can force entry of potassium back into the cell. Calcium gluconate decreases neuromuscular irritability by stabilizing the cellular membrane. Sodium bicarbonate corrects acid-base disorders by forcing potassium back into the cell.

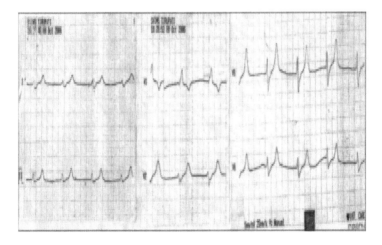

Calcium concentration is normally 2.2 – 2.6 mmol/L. Cardiac muscles require extracellular calcium ions for contraction. An influx of calcium into the cell sustains depolarization and muscle contraction, as well as relaxation. Nerve conduction throughout the heart is facilitated by calcium. Calcium also helps to maintain the cell membrane integrity by establishing an action potential.

Hypocalcemia can be caused by pancreatitis, diuretics, hypoparathyroidism, blood transfusions, metabolic or respiratory alkalosis, and vitamin D deficiency. The EKG will most predominantly reflect a **prolonged QT-interval**. Hypocalcemia creates increased neuromuscular excitability, which causes partial depolarization of muscle cells. As a result, reduced stimulus is required to initiate an action potential. This causes prolonged ventricular depolarization and decreased cardiac contractility. Severe symptoms can range from seizures and tetany to respiratory arrest and death. Treatment should include IV replacement with calcium gluconate and avoiding phosphate intake, as they have an inverse relationship.

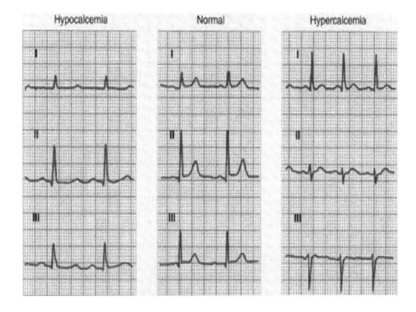

Hypercalcemia can be asymptomatic, but increased calcium can often be the result of other diseases. It can be caused by excessive skeletal calcium release, malignancies, increased intestinal calcium absorption, decreased calcium excretion, adrenal insufficiency, hyperparathyroidism, or thyrotoxicosis. Symptoms are the result of an increased threshold for depolarization resulting in a general slowing of body processes. The mnemonic "Stones, Bones, Groans, Thrones, & Psych Overtones" describes renal or biliary symptoms, bone pain, abdominal pain, polyuria or **Osborn waves** (looks like additional R-wave), and insomnia or coma. Hypercalcemia has a negative chronotropic effect, decreasing the heart rate. This results in a **shortened QT-interval**. Interventions for hypercalcemia include loop diuretics, synthetic calcitonin, IV normal saline, oral fluids, phosphate, and decreased dietary intake.

MEDICATIONS

Class I-A: Quinidine, Procainamide, & Disopyramide are fast Na-channel blockers used for ventricular arrhythmias. These medications cause prolongation of the QRS and QT-interval. They may also cause Torsades de Pointes (polymorphic ventricular tachycardia).

Class I-B: Lidocaine, Tocainide, Mexiletine, & Phenytoin are Na-channel blockers used for ventricular tachycardia and treatment & prevention during & immediately after myocardial infarction. They have little effect on the EKG but may cause a slight prolongation of QRS in an overdose.

Class I-C: Flecainide, Propafenone, & Moricizine are Na-channel blockers used to prevent atrial fibrillation and treat recurrent tachyarrhythmias. They can prolong the PR-interval & QRS and can precipitate ventricular tachycardia.

Class II Beta-blockers: Propranolol, Metoprolol, & Esmolol block beta-receptors and are used to decrease MI mortality and prevent tachyarrhythmias. They can cause profound bradycardia.

Class III: Amiodarone, Sotalol, & Ibutilide are K-channel blockers (Amiodarone has Class I, II, III, & IV activity, Sotalol is a BB) used in WPW syndrome, ventricular tachycardia (sotalol), and atrial flutter/fibrillation (ibutilide). They can prolong the QT-interval and can lead to Torsades de Pointes.

Calcium Channel Blockers: Verapamil, Diltiazem, & Nicardipine attenuate the influx of calcium into the cell thereby reducing contraction of arteries (alleviating hypertension), force of contraction, and speed of electrical conduction. They can slow conduction through the AV-node creating an AV block or create severe bradycardia.

Digitalis is used in heart failure to increase contractility by inhibiting Na/K ATPase pumps in the myocardial cells. It also slows conduction through the AV node. Digitalis can **depress the ST-segment**, flatten T-waves, prolong PR-intervals, shorten QT-intervals, and dysrhythmias can occur with toxicity.

Adenosine slows conduction through the AV node and interrupts AV re-entry pathways. It is used to treat supraventricular tachycardia (SVT). It has a very short half-life and must, therefor, be flushed immediately to reach the heart before being metabolized within seconds. At the time of conversion to sinus rhythm, several new rhythms may appear including hearts blocks, asystole, and ventricular fibrillation. The rhythms are typically transient and resolve quickly.

When beginning the initial administration of antidysrhythmics or caring for a patient on antidysrhythmics, document QRS and QT-intervals, observe for desired effects, and observe for and report adverse effects.

CHAPTER 6. PUTTING IT TOGETHER

Using a systematic approach to interpreting EKG's is important so that vital characteristics are not overlooked. Features that require analysis include heart rate, rhythm, intervals, conduction defects, chamber enlargement, and ST & T-wave changes. This section will provide a step-by-step guide regarding how to evaluate each of these features.

COMPONENTS

Heart rate can be calculated easily if the rhythm is regular by counting the number of 1 mm squares between two heart beats (RR-interval) and dividing this number into 3000 if the paper speed is 50 mm/s (3000 = 1 minute b/c 60 sec. x 50 = 3000), or into 1500 if the paper speed is 25 mm/s (the common standard). If the heart rate is irregular, the average over a period of time must be determined. It is important to note that 30 large squares or 150 mm represent 3 seconds at 50 mm/s or 6 seconds at 25 mm/s. The heart rate can be evaluated by counting the number of QRS complexes over 30 large squares and multiplying by 20 if at 50 mm/s or 10 if at 25 mm/s. Conventionally, a normal heart rate is 60 – 100 bpm. Clinical context is important because a well-trained athlete, for example, may have a heart rate of 85 bpm, which should be considered tachycardia.

Rhythm refers to the pattern that the heart beats and the electrical sequence displayed on EKG. Determining the heart rhythm requires evaluation of:

- Regularity of heart beats by viewing R-to-R intervals (Sinus Arrhythmia, A-Fib, V-Fib)

P-Waves represent atrial depolarization and in a normal EKG, the P-wave should precede the QRS complex. The amplitude is normally 0.05 – 0.25 mV (0.5 – 2.5 small boxes) and duration should be 0.04 – 0.11 seconds (1 – 3 small boxes). The shape is usually smooth and rounded.

- Presence or absence of P-wave before every QRS (PAC, A-fib)

- P-wave height > 2.5 mm in lead II or V1 (RAH)

- P-wave duration > 0.12 in lead II (LAH, PAC)

- Regularity of P-P intervals, observe pattern (Blocks)

- Presence of QRS following every P-wave (2nd, 3rd degree blocks)

- Are they smooth, rounded, and similar (RAH)

- P-wave inversion (Junctional, LAH)

PR-Interval indicates AV conduction time. Measure the interval from beginning of P-wave to beginning of QRS complex. The interval is typically 0.12 – 0.20 seconds (3 – 5 small boxes). Remember that the interval shortens with increased heart rate. They should be constant in length.

- PR-interval length 0.12 – 0.20 seconds (1st, 2nd degree block, Junctional, WPW)

- PR-interval constant across entire tracing (2nd, 3rd degree blocks)

- PR-segment depression (Pericarditis)

QRS Complex reflects ventricular depolarization, which causes a mechanical contraction. The QRS usually consists of three wave components. The length should be 0.04 – 0.12 seconds (1 to 3 small boxes).

- QRS length is 0.04 – 0.12 seconds (SVT, BBB, PVC, Junctional, V-Tach)

- QRS complexes are similar in appearance (PVC, WPW, Ventricular Pacing, LVH, RVH)

- QRS widened (BBB, Hyperkalemia, Paced, WPW)

T-Wave reflects repolarization of the ventricles and is asymmetrical following the QRS complex. The T-wave may be deflected downward or appear tall and peaked. A U-wave is a small, upright bump directly following the T-wave.

- T-wave upright or tall & peaked (Hyper-K, STEMI)

- T-wave inverted (Ischemia, Infarct, PE, ICP, BBB, LVH, RVH)

- U-wave present (Hypo-K)

QT-Interval reflects the time of ventricular depolarization and repolarization. It is measured from the beginning of the QRS complex to the end of the T-wave. The QT-interval is 0.36 – 0.44 seconds (9 – 11 small boxes). QT-intervals vary with heart rate. Normally, the QT-interval is less than half the R-R-interval if normal sinus rhythm.

- QT-interval 0.36 – 0.44 seconds (lengthened = Hypo-K, Hypo-Ca, Hypo-Mg, MI, Ischemia, ICP, Meds, Hypothermia)

- QT-interval less than ½ R-R interval (short QT syndrome is genetic and found in young adults, may lead to sudden cardiac arrest in otherwise healthy pt)

ST-Segment reflects the early repolarization of the ventricles. It extends from the end of the QRS to the beginning of the T-wave and is normally isoelectric.

- ST-segment elevation (Acute MI, Pericarditis, LBBB, LVH, ICP)

- ST-segment depression (Ischemia/NSTEMI, Posterior MI, Digoxin, Hypo-K, SVT, RBBB, RVH, LBBB, LVH)

Q-Wave is any negative deflection that precedes an R-wave. It represents the normal left-to-right depolarization of the Intraventricular septum. Small Q-waves are normal.

- Q-wave deeper than 2 mm in V1 – 3 (MI)

APPROACH

1. Trust your first impression.

- Examine the EKG briefly and see what jumps out. Often times, pacer spikes, peak T-wave, or other prominent findings can be very telling. Retain this first impression before methodically narrowing your search. Keep it in mind moving forward.

2. Explore it piecemeal and in detail.

- Consider each beat and determine if and how they look different from one another. Use the normal beats and their segments, intervals, etc. as comparison. Do you see PVC's, bundle branch blocks, or anything abnormal?

3. Rate?

- Tachy/brady, irregular/regular?

4. Rhythm?

- Irregular/regular, P-waves present and uniform, P-to-QRS ratio, complexes, intervals, wide/narrow, depressed, peaked,   notched?

5. Hypertrophy?

- LAH, RAH, LVH, RVH, strain patterns?

6. Ischemia or Infarct?

- T-wave & ST-segment abnormalities, Q-waves?

7. List.

- Record rate, rhythm, hypertrophy, intervals deviations, blocks, and ST & T-wave deviations.

8. Correlate.

- Are there any physical findings or otherwise that support my impression?

CONCLUSION

As you have seen, without a regular rate and rhythm, the heart will not be able to efficiently pump and circulate oxygenated blood and other nutrients to the tissues and organs of the body. Hopefully, the critical nature of this topic has been impressed upon the reader. We have reviewed each phase of the cardiac cycle and how these are reflected by specific waveforms within the EKG. The major dysrhythmias have been identified along with multiple causative factors. Moving forward, this book should serve as a guide to accurately analyze the important information that the EKG offers concerning the electrical activity of the heart.

The nurse should, at this point, be capable of analyzing the EKG in a systematic manner to determine the patient's cardiac rhythm and to detect dysrhythmias and conduction disorders, as well as evidence of myocardial ischemia, injury, and infarction. Once the rhythm has been analyzed, the findings should be compared with and matched to the EKG criteria put forth in this book to assist with a differential diagnosis. It is important for the nurse to assess the patient to determine the physiologic effects of the dysrhythmia and to identify possible causes. Treatment of dysrhythmias is based on the etiology and the effect of the dysrhythmia, not on its presence alone.

An EKG is often the initial component of diagnostic testing available in the evaluation of a patient. A proper understanding of the EKG allows early detection of important pathological and physiological issues. Early intervention is the key and a skilled nurse uses the EKG in many situations to gain insight into their patients' status.

A comprehensive understanding is crucial and we hope that you will continue to develop your understanding of electrophysiology by viewing and analyzing as many strips as possible. We encourage you to make it a point to seek out real-life examples within your clinical setting. Repetition is the key to successful understanding. Gather all information at your disposal and trust yourself when you are interpreting an EKG.

ABOUT THE AUTHOR

I started as a Respiratory Therapist in Kansas City, Missouri before attending Baker University in Kansas for undergraduate nursing. My first job was in the medical ICU at the University of Colorado Hospital. After practicing for several years I decided to attend the University of Pennsylvania in Philadelphia for Nurse Anesthesia School. I have practiced Nurse Anesthesia in both North Carolina and the Chicago area. I have taught nursing school, performed nursing NCLEX board symposiums, and practiced Nurse Anesthesia.

My wife, Kristin, and I enjoy endurance sports, volunteering abroad, and backpacking in Colorado. Kristin attended Baker & Penn with me and has practiced at UCH as well as North Carolina. We love education and strive to share what we know.

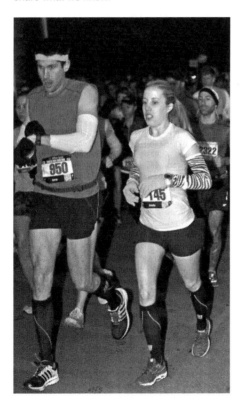

DISCLAIMER

As with all forms of science, nursing is a work in progress. What is taken as common knowledge today, may well be proven wrong tomorrow. Such is the nature of the scientific process. With this in mind, we stress that the information contained in this book is for the sole purpose of preparing for and mastering nursing board examinations. The information has been thoroughly reviewed and put forth with the intention of disseminating up to date knowledge and known best practices at the time of publishing. The content is not intended as a substitute for the medical advice of physicians or proper nursing training. Given the nature of this subject matter, we cannot guarantee the absence of error or promise scholastic success or clinical aptitude. All contents of this book are not to be construed as endorsements of practice or prescribed therapy for any specific clinical situation. The information reflects the author's, publisher's, and all other involved party's understanding of study strategies regarding registered nursing didactic application.

We abjure any responsibility of incorrect content, consequences of enacting therapies contained within, liability to any party for any loss, damage, or disruption caused by errors or omissions, whether such errors or omissions result from negligence, accident, or any other cause. We encourage the reader to clarify any points with outside sources and consult the national standards according to your profession's governing practice body.

Printed in Great Britain
by Amazon